THIS NOTEBOOK BELONGS TO

____

Made in the USA
Las Vegas, NV
02 September 2021

29444587R00069